I0429045

30-Day Whole Food Cleanse

Plant Based Whole Foods for Beginners

Jason Kayne

Table of Contents

Strawberry-Beet Smoothie

Veggie Breakfast Bowl

Banana Breakfast Cookies

Fig Smoothie

Baked Fruity Oatmeal

LUNCH RECIPES

Potato Soup

Oven Baked Mexican Bean Burgers

Portabella "Steaks" And Veggies

White Bean-Quinoa Lunch Salad

String Beans With Sesame

Veggie Slow Cooker Goulas

Squash And Coconut Slow-Cooker Curry

Yellow Split Pea Stew

Oven Baked Cauliflower Steaks

Green Beans And Pine Nuts

Rice and Bean Casserole

Roasted Lunch Bowl

Falafel Wrap

Bean And Vegetable Chili

Quinoa Stuffed Tomatoes

Bean Bites

Broccoli Soup

Vegetable Stew

Quinoa Curry Bowl

Rainbow Burgers

Veggie Based Loaf

DINNER RECIPES

Mediterranean Couscous

Sweet Potato Burgers

Red Lentil Curry

"Meatballs" Without Meat

Spring Quinoa

Lettuce Wraps

Veggie Pizza

Rice and Tahini Cakes

Cauliflower Rice With Zucchinis

Soy Beans Salad With Asparagus And Dill

Soy Bean And Spinach Slow-Cooker Enchiladas

Braised Cabbage with Raisins

Spicy Tomato and Basil Soup

Curry Zucchini Soup

Introduction

For many of us, part of our New Year's resolutions often includes such things like: 'be healthy', 'lose more weight', 'get a slender body', 'eat the right foods', or any other goal similar to these that revolves around eating healthy and being physically fit. If your resolution happens to fall in this category, you are not alone; millions of others have a similar goal.

But while many of us have such wishes, we somehow never seem to achieve whatever it is we want. Then the question that you may ask is; why do you always seem to give up on your goals? Well, one reason why many of us give up is simply because we follow extreme diets that are just unsustainable in the long term.

We adopt diets hoping to shed weight after a few days then go back to our unhealthy eating habits. And when that happens, we start putting back all the weight that we had lost. Besides, adopting some of these highly restrictive diets is unhealthy because they limit our intake of essential nutrients. So when we realize that we are putting on weight and experiencing the negative effects of eating nutrient-restricted diets, we give up.

Well, that doesn't have to be you; you can adopt a healthy whole food diet that you can easily take for the rest of your life. The good thing with such a diet is that you don't feel restricted because you eat healthy, nutrient-dense foods that enhance your overall health. And besides, when you lose weight, even over the long term, you can be sure that you won't put on the weight back because you don't have to stop taking whole foods; you can follow the diet for the rest of your life.

This book has comprehensive information that will help you understand how to follow a whole foods plant based diet plan for up to 30 days. You can replicate the information you will learn from this book to follow the diet for the rest of your life. To ensure that you have a smooth time, the book also provides over 50 delicious recipes that you can prepare at home.

Chapter 1: Plant Based Whole Foods: An Overview

For many of us, our food mostly comprises of meat and dairy products, which is good because these foods do contain the proteins, carbohydrates and good fats our body requires to function well. However, we focus so much on what benefits these foods can provide us with that we ignore that consuming too much of these foods can expose us to various problems. For instance, the high intake of these foods increases the glucose and fat levels in our bodies, thus slowly increasing our chances of developing health problems such as hypertension, diabetes, and heart conditions. This is especially so when you combine our high protein, carbohydrates and fats intake with the fact that many of these foods contain traces of different chemicals that could end up causing lots of other complications given that they cause high levels of toxicity within our bodies. Too much exposure to some of these chemicals and genetically modified versions of various foods could result to toxins build up, which may in turn trigger the development of some of the health conditions mentioned above. This is also worsened by our intake of highly processed foods since these often contain preservatives, additives, colorings, and many other chemicals that only end up increasing our likelihood of suffering from some of these health conditions.

So what can you do to minimize the likelihood of suffering from some of these health complications? Well, the answer to this is simple; replace your processed, non-organic foods with organic food sources. This is what constitutes a whole foods diet. So what exactly is a whole food diet?

What is a Whole Food Diet?

In its simplest terms, a whole food diet simply refers to a diet consisting of food, which still looks as it does when it is growing in nature or is just very close to its original shape. So in essence, this means food that hasn't been messed up with or has simply been minimally messed with. Everything (i.e. fiber and the nutrients) within the whole vegetable, nut, legume, grain, seed, or fruit is still intact. And with that kind of food, the body is able to run efficiently in its natural form or very close to it. So when you consider a plant based whole food diet (also referred to as a vegan diet), this simply entails taking plant based whole foods.

Since it is plant based, you won't be eating dairy, eggs and meat. Such food has to be as close to its natural form as possible although minimal processing is often allowed. For instance, minimal processing could entail making applesauce from apples, making a green smoothie from kale and fruit, making carrot juice from carrots or making pancakes using oat flour after grounding rolled oats. As you process, you have to make sure that you take GMO free ingredients. A whole food diet is centered entirely on eating unrefined (or at times minimally refined) and unprocessed whole plant based foods. What you expect to eat includes vegetables, fruits, whole grains, legumes, and tubers.

Processed foods like refined sugar, oil, and bleached flour are not allowed. However, it is not mandatory that you completely stop eating these foods. You can restrict your intake of these foods and keep them to a minimum. This way, you won't feel that you are banned from eating your favorite steak or the poached egg you often crave for. You can still indulge in these little pleasures while following the plant and whole food based diet and stay perfectly healthy at the same time.

Think about it; we are hard wired (by evolution) to digest and utilize the foods that were readily available long before the industrial revolution. In fact, our body is still in its 'paleolithic' form despite the tremendous milestones that we've made in different aspects of our lives. Unfortunately, when we take foods that the body hasn't yet evolved to digest and assimilate, the body simply treats these as foreign bodies (or just toxins), which it stores or finds ways of eliminating. For instance, when you eat oily salty potato chips, your body has to work harder to eliminate toxins from the fats and other components within the food that are just not healthy for us. Much of the food we eat today goes through manufacturing, refining, or processing where such ingredients like sugar, oil, salt and other chemicals and preservatives are added while others like water and fiber are removed. As I already stated, this often triggers a response by the body to remove any toxins within such foods. The process ultimately results to a wide array of complications. So how does the diet work?

How The Diet Works?

The diet is largely based on the principle that whole foods (plants based) contain the perfect balance of nutrients your body needs and can help you stay fit, healthy, and beautiful. For instance, such foods contain all sorts of vitamins, proteins, carbohydrates, trace minerals, fiber, water and even the good fats needed for the proper and healthy functioning of your body. So when you slowly shift to a whole foods based diet, you won't be depriving your body of healthy nutrients. Instead, you'll be giving it precisely what it needs. In fact, as I already explained, our body has evolved (and hardwired itself) to process such foods efficiently so you can be sure that such foods won't cause toxicity.

Secondly, whole foods easily travel down your gut and aren't difficult to break down. This can make the digestion process smoother and easier. And with an improved digestion, such problems like heartburn, diarrhea, acidity and several other similar issues will be gone when you take whole plant based foods. And with an improved digestion, you will start noticing an improvement in your health.

Another notable feature of a whole foods diet is the fact that it eliminates processed foods that are often very high in calories derived from added sugar and fat. Eating highly processed and high calorie foods can easily make you gain weight especially because such foods lack fiber and are rich in simple sugars, which the body breaks down very fast thus leaving you craving for more after a short period. The high calorie content coupled with the fact that such foods are digested fast means that you are likely to eat more of these, which in turn means that you will probably end up with a calorie surplus, thus increasing your chances of gaining weight. Whole foods are satiating due to their dietary fiber, which means that they take a lot of time before they can be eliminated from the body or before the body can signal you to take more food. Besides, they are rich in complex carbohydrates, which are also broken down slowly so the likelihood of overeating such foods is small. And as such, it is easy to limit your calorie consumption even if you are not counting calories especially because you end up eating less.

Note: Unlike many diet books out there, a whole foods diet plan does not require any calorie counting, supplements or complicated meal plans especially because it is pretty much straight forward; all you have to do is to restrict your intake of processed foods then eat mainly whole foods or those that are close to their natural state as possible.

So what is it you can eat while on this diet? That's what we will discuss in the next chapter.

Chapter 2: What to Eat and What Not to Eat in this Diet

Contrary to what you may have thought, a plant-based diet is not just taking leafy vegetables like kale, spinach, and collard greens every single day. You can take many more foods including starchy vegetables and fruits. Let's discuss this in detail to help you understand the variety of foods that you can take:

Foods You Can Eat

You are completely allowed to eat all the following foods while on a plant based whole food diet.

• Fruit: You can eat any unprocessed organic fruit you like when following this diet. You are allowed to eat grapes, berries, bananas, apples, mangoes, oranges, avocado, kiwi and every fruit that falls in the category.

• Vegetables: All organic unprocessed vegetables are allowed in this diet. Make sure to eat lettuce, spinach, broccoli, collard green, cauliflower, carrots, kale and cabbage as these veggies are rich in antioxidants and vitamins that are essential for your body.

• Legumes: You can eat chickpeas, lima beans, lentils, kidney beans, black beans, cannellini beans and other beans that fall in the 'legumes' category.

• Whole Grains: All the whole grains, including rice, barley, oats, whole wheat, quinoa and millet are allowed in this diet. Note that protein from wheat is not good if you are gluten intolerant.

• Starchy Veggies and Tubers: You are allowed to eat starchy veggies like potatoes when on this diet. In this case, you can eat yams, winter squash, green peas, yucca, corn and other starchy veggies and tubers as well.

• Seeds and Nuts: You can eat all types of seeds and nuts, including walnuts, almonds, cashew nuts, pecan, hemp seeds, flax seeds, chia seeds and sunflower seeds.

• Soy, Almond and Coconut Milk: You can add these different types of milk to your diet, but try limiting their intake.

Note: Insist on eating organic unprocessed foods. You can find these from your local groceries market. In fact, get these foods from your local farmers market as opposed to the grocery store.

So what is it that you should not eat while on a plant based whole food diet? Let's discuss this briefly:

Foods You Must Not Consume

• Processed Foods: You must not eat processed and refined foods that mostly come in the form of packaged foods.

• Frozen and Ready-to-cook Meals: You aren't allowed to eat ready-to-cook or frozen meals when following this diet as they are rich in trans-fat and artificial ingredients.

• Foods Packed with Calories and Harmful Ingredients: You must read the nutritional information when buying any foods and other ingredients just to ensure that you are eating healthy foods.

You are not allowed to eat meat, including beef, pork, mutton, chicken and seafood as well as milk and dairy products, eggs and pasta in the diet. However, experts suggest you don't completely eliminate these foods from your diet, so you don't feel suffocated. If you have to eat them, only eat them once or maybe twice a week but not more than that to ensure that you don't end up spiking your blood sugar and fat levels. If you can eliminate their consumption, then that is amazing.

Tips to remember:

Limit your salt and sugar intake greatly. Although you are allowed to add salt and sugar to your recipes, make sure it does not go beyond ½ to 1 teaspoon per 4 servings.

In addition, you should try limiting your use of processed oil or fat while on this diet. Instead, you can take olive, coconut and other vegetable oils, but try limiting their intake. Other sources of fats and oils include avocados, canola, nuts (mentioned above) etc.

And when you adopt such a diet, you can still be sure that you will derive a wide array of benefits including the ones we are going to discuss in the next chapter.

Chapter 3: Benefits of Following this Diet

By now, you do have some idea of why this diet is good for you. Let us build up on this to help you understand more on how you stand to gain by adopting a whole foods diet.

Prevents heart problems

A recent study conducted on 400,000 Europeans proved that taking a diet that is largely plant based (even 70 percent plant based is enough) can lower your risk of suffering from cardiovascular disease by up to 20%. And why is that so?

Well, a plant based whole food diet containing such ingredients as legumes, whole grains, vegetables, fruit, beans and others is likely to have low levels of saturated fat (found in meat and animal products) and trans fats. Saturated fats have been linked with increased amounts of cholesterol in the blood, which in turn increases the risk of stroke and heart attack.

In addition, when you are on a plant-based diet, it is easy to limit your cholesterol intake. In particular, if you avoid foods high in bad cholesterol (HDL), this makes it easy to avoid plaque buildup. The plaque is also made up of fat, calcium and other waste products. And when it builds up within the arteries (carry blood away from your heart), this can actually cause them to block and even harden resulting to the risk of strokes or heart attacks. When you go on a plant based diet, you are able to replace saturated fats and oils with polyunsaturated and/or monounsaturated fats (often found in such foods like nuts, olive oil, and avocadoes). Keep in mind that less than 10% of your daily calories intake should come from saturated fats. A plant based diet is also likely to be high in phytochemicals and plant sterols that help break down cholesterol and fat quickly and easily. It is also high in potassium which helps control sodium levels in the body thus ultimately controls hypertension. Some foods high in potassium include soybeans, mushrooms, apricots, bananas, spinach, sweet potatoes and cantaloupe.

When you go on a plant-based diet, you can easily increase your intake of soluble fiber, which is one of the ways through which you can reduce bad cholesterol from circulating in your body. Additionally, the soluble fiber acts on the bad cholesterol within your gut and helps get rid of it more quickly from your body, which in turn lowers the overall amount of bad cholesterol that your body absorbs. You can get soluble fiber from lentils, nuts, veggies, fruits, beans etc.

The consumption of meat or high saturated fat has been linked with a high risk of suffering from type 2 diabetes. And when you suffer from diabetes, you almost double your likelihood of suffering from heart disease and stroke. As for weight loss, you reduce your saturated fat intake when you lose weight while on a plant based diet. We will discuss more on how a plant based diet links to weight loss.

By reducing your intake of meat and processed foods (which are often high in sodium), along with other animal products, you can reduce your likelihood of suffering from hypertension.

Plant based foods are often high in omega 3 fatty acids, which have been noted to reduce your risk of heart disease, diabetes, hypertension and cholesterol. You can take such foods like canola oil, flaxseeds, walnuts, pumpkin seeds, and soybeans to get sufficient amounts of omega 3s.

Weight loss

A plant based whole food diet is likely to constitute components that have properties that facilitate weight loss. Here are some of these properties:

It is likely to be high in soluble fiber. Fiber slows down the digestion process and since fiber itself is not digested, this means that you are likely to feel full for longer. This in turn helps you to reduce your intake of food and subsequently lowering your calorie intake. This of course is bound to make it easier for you to create the much desired calorie deficit.

The diet is rich in complex carbohydrates, which are generally metabolized at a slower rate than the simple carbohydrates often found in processed foods. This simply means that you are likely to experience stable blood sugar levels and the likelihood of having to eat to satisfy your cravings is reduced.

Taking a plant based whole food diet high in raw clean whole foods may actually increase your chances of losing weight. This is especially so because such a diet is likely to be high in water content (which is filling and low in calories), minerals and vitamins. The good thing about the diet is that you don't even feel deprived or have to go hungry, which means following it is very easy.

A plant based whole food diet is likely to help you to fight constipation, which can in turn help you to avoid inflammation, which can in turn help you to minimize weight loss related to inflammation.

In this diet, you are avoiding your intake of highly processed foods filled with added sugars and other high calorie ingredients. As such, your calories intake is bound to reduce drastically while on this diet thus making it easier for you to lose weight. When you couple this with the fact that pound for pound, plant based foods are often lower in calories than meat and animal based foods, this means that you are likely to be taking lesser calories while on a plant based diet.

It can help you fight or prevent diabetes

For starters, a plant-based diet can help you to manage your blood sugar levels especially because of the high complex carbohydrates content in such foods. Unlike simple carbohydrates, complex carbohydrates are broken down slowly, which simply means that you are unlikely to notice drastic increases and reductions in your blood sugar levels. Subsequently, you are unlikely to experience spikes in your insulin levels, which often leads to insulin resistance, a precursor to diabetes. The diet also fights diabetes due to its high fiber, high plant protein, high antioxidant, and low cholesterol content. Plant based foods help allow insulin to enter the bloodstream at a slower rate, which in turn helps to manage blood glucose more efficiently.

Other benefits of a whole foods-plant based diet include fighting constipation, improving skin health, reducing your likelihood of suffering from cancer, boosting your energy, improving sleep and reducing inflammation.

If these benefits give you some motivation to start following a whole foods plant based diet, let's get to the specifics of following the diet plan. We will learn all that in the next chapters. How can you implement this diet plan? Well, to help you understand how to follow the diet, I will break this up into a 4 weeks diet, which will ultimately help you to achieve the benefits we've just talked about.

Chapter 4: 30 Days Guide To Plant Based Whole Food Diet

Now that you know what you can and what you cannot eat in this diet as well as understand the benefits of this diet, let's now try to learn how to go on this diet plan.

Week 1

The first week is all about getting started, preparing your mind and body for this big change and slowly easing into the diet regimen, which is why you won't be making any dynamic shifts to your diet in this week.

As a beginner, you need to pace yourself and gradually move towards making big changes to your diet because if you instantly stop consuming meat, dairy, and eggs, and try eating vegetables and legumes, you will soon lose motivation and will quit for good.

Note:

1: Studies show that people who make gradual healthy changes to their diet are able to stick to it for a longer time as compared to those who quit unhealthy foods cold turkey. This is why it is essential to go slow and steady because this is how you win a race.

2: About cheat meals and animal based meals: I know that I have mentioned that while on this diet, you are not to take animal products. Well, while this is completely true, I want you to ease into the diet plan. That's why I am making provisions for animal based meals.

3: You can refer to the recipes section to know how to make some of these meals.

Tip: You need to have a notebook where you write everything related to this diet. Make an entry in the diary daily to help you know what you are eating and how you're feeling. This will help you track your performance and understand the amazing effects that this diet has on your mind and body.

To make the adjustment easy for you, here's a seven day breakup of the first week so you can make healthy adjustments while on this diet.

MONDAY

Breakfast: 1 glass milk + one apple

Lunch: 1 bowl of potato soup+ fresh fruit

Dinner: Beef chili and rice

TUESDAY

Breakfast: ½ bowl quinoa and fruits + 2 boiled eggs

Lunch: 1 bowl of green salad + 2 pieces fried chicken

Dinner: 200g of steak + 1 bowl of red lentil curry

WEDNESDAY

Breakfast: Apple Pecan Smoothie + 1 seasonal fruit + ½ glass milk

Lunch: Portabella steaks and veggies + fig smoothie + 100g of beef (any recipe you like)

Dinner: 150g of steak + one sweet potato burger

THURSDAY:

Breakfast: Breakfast savory cakes + blueberry smoothie + 1 egg

Lunch: Oven baked Mexican bean burgers + a piece of fried chicken

Dinner: Quinoa curry bowl

FRIDAY

Breakfast: Banana muffins + ½ glass of milk

Lunch: Yellow split pea stew

Dinner: Veggie pizza + 1 bowl tomato and basil soup

SATURDAY

Breakfast: Chickpea omelet + strawberry beet smoothie

Lunch: Bean and vegetable chili + one breakfast savory cake

Dinner: Mediterranean Couscous + 2 lettuce wraps

SUNDAY

Breakfast: Banana pancakes + strawberry beet smoothie

Lunch: Lunch of your choice (can contain meat) + vegetable salad

Dinner: Cheat meal (eat anything you want)

Tip: Try to reward yourself as well. You can buy yourself something nice like a pair of shoes, clothes etc or watch a movie to celebrate your progress.

Week 2

If week one went smoothly, you'll be able to adjust easily into the second week.

The second week is about bidding farewell to dairy products and eggs. Here's a breakup of the week to make it easy for you to implement such changes into your diet.

Tip: Make sure to eat a handful of nuts or sip your favorite nutritious smoothie if any of the signs of detoxification bother you

MONDAY

Breakfast: 1 egg + potato oven pancakes

Lunch: 1 big bowl of salad+ 1 fruit

Dinner: Rice and tahini cakes + green salad + Mediterranean couscous

TUESDAY

Breakfast: 1 egg + apple pecan smoothie + 1 banana pancake

Lunch: White bean quinoa lunch salad + fresh fruit

Dinner: Cauliflower rice with zucchini + creamy curried cauliflower soup

WEDNESDAY

Breakfast: Apple Pecan Smoothie + 1 glass of milk + 1 egg

Lunch: Portabella steaks and veggies + fruit salad

Dinner: Soy bean and spinach slow cooker

THURSDAY

Breakfast: Breakfast savory cakes + blueberry smoothie

Lunch: Rice and bean casserole

Dinner: Veggie based loaf + red lentil curry

FRIDAY

Breakfast: Fruity bowl + strawberry beet smoothie

Lunch: Squash and coconut slow cooker curry

Dinner: Spring quinoa + fresh fruit platter

SATURDAY

Breakfast: Apple and cinnamon oatmeal squares

Lunch: Green pea guacamole wrap + fresh fruit salad

Dinner: Black bean and rice

SUNDAY

Breakfast: Hot cereal with dried fruits + strawberry beet smoothie

Lunch: Spinach salad + lentil chili

Dinner: Whole grain pasta with lots of green veggies and beans

Tip: Don't forget to review your log, so you can know how well you have been doing.

Week 3

The third week is going to bring a big change in your diet, so it's going to be a little challenging for you, but you can do it. If you have been good to your body for two weeks, you can certainly offer it a lot more.

The third week is about taking things up a notch. By now, meat, eggs and dairy will almost be eliminated entirely from your diet and you are going to focus on eating whole foods only. Here's what you need to do on the seven days of this week to come closer to reaching your goal of becoming healthy and fit.

MONDAY

Breakfast: Green salad with strawberries and apples

Lunch: Grilled herb seasoned turkey + green salad

Dinner: Grilled shrimp and veggie kebabs + vegetable confetti cauliflower rice

TUESDAY

Breakfast: English muffin + banana and strawberry smoothie

Lunch: Garbanzo and veggie stuffed pita + fruit salad

Dinner Soy bean salad with asparagus and dill + tomato soup

WEDNESDAY

Breakfast: Apple Pecan Smoothie + baked fruity oatmeal

Lunch: Broccoli soup+ fresh fruit

Dinner: Soy bean salad with asparagus and dill + tomato soup

THURSDAY

Breakfast: Banana breakfast cookies + blueberry smoothie

Lunch: Rainbow burgers + banana muffin

Dinner: String beans with sesame + red lentil curry

FRIDAY

Breakfast: Apple and cinnamon oatmeal squares + spinach, kale and beet smoothie

Lunch: Veggie slow cooker goulash + fresh fruit

Dinner: Green beans and pine nuts + fresh fruit platter

SATURDAY

Breakfast: Garden salad with cabbage, apple and berries

Lunch: Oven baked cauliflower steaks + apple and orange smoothie

Dinner: Braised cabbage with raisins + 1 bowl tomato and basil soup

SUNDAY

Breakfast: Banana pancakes + strawberry beet smoothie

Lunch: Spinach salad + fresh fruit

Dinner: 2 slices Veggie pizza + ½ bowl spring quinoa

Tip: Like every last day of the previous two weeks, this day is going to be a treat day. Do something exciting today to appreciate yourself for the amazing changes you have made to your diet.

Week 4

The last week is not going to bring any drastic change in your diet, since you have already done that in the previous three weeks. Let us look at what you should do on the seven days of the fourth week.

MONDAY

Breakfast: Hot cereal with strawberry and banana smoothie

Lunch: Bulgur with roasted tomatoes, asparagus and balsamic vinegar

Dinner: Baked tortilla chips + homemade salsa and lentil chili

TUESDAY

Breakfast: Quinoa fruity bowl

Lunch: Salmon and greens with quinoa + fruit salad

Dinner: Carrot and cashew spread and celery sticks + red lentil curry

WEDNESDAY

Breakfast: Apple Pecan Smoothie + baked fruity oatmeal

Lunch: Hummus and roasted veggie wraps + fresh fruit

Dinner: Soy bean salad with asparagus and dill + tomato soup

THURSDAY

Breakfast: Banana breakfast cookies + blueberry smoothie

Lunch: Whole grain wrap containing black bean salad and avocado-lime dressing

Dinner: Soba noodles with carrots and green veggies

FRIDAY

Breakfast: Cauliflower scramble + spinach, kale and beet smoothie

Lunch: Lentil chili with brown rice + fresh fruit

Dinner: Green beans and pine nuts + fresh fruit platter

SATURDAY

Breakfast: Garden salad with cabbage, apple and berries + orange, strawberry and banana smoothie

Lunch: Whole wheat pasta with kale and carrots

Dinner: Meatballs without meatball + 1 bowl tomato and basil soup

SUNDAY

Breakfast: Quinoa fruity bowl + strawberry beet smoothie

Lunch: Vegetable stew + fresh fruit

Dinner: Cauliflower rice with zucchinis

Delicious Plant Based Whole Food Recipes

Breakfast Recipes

Chickpea "Omelet"

Serves: 4
Time: 15 minutes

Ingredients:

1 cup chickpea flour
1/3 cup nutritional yeast
½ teaspoon onion powder
½ teaspoon garlic powder
2 green onions, chopped
1 avocado, peeled, stoned
¼ teaspoon black pepper
1 cup water

Directions:

In a bowl, combine the chickpea flour, onion powder, garlic powder, yeast, and black pepper. Add water and stir until smooth.

Heat non-stick skillet over medium-high heat; pour in the batter, like making pancakes and sprinkle with green onions. Once the bottom is browned flip the omelet. Cook for 1-2 minutes more and serve. Top with sliced avocado.

Banana Oats

Serves: 4
Time: 20 minutes

Ingredients:

2 cups oats
1 banana, sliced
½ cup almonds, silvered
½ cup dates, pitted
½ cup water
1 cup of almond milk

Directions:

Preheat oven to 275F and line baking sheet with parchment paper.

Place the dates in saucepan and cover with water. Cook for 10 minutes over medium heat.

Remove from the heat and place in food blender. Add the banana and process until smooth.

Add the oats and almonds to the mixture and spread over baking sheet; bake for 40 minutes stirring every 10 minutes.

Remove from the oven and place in a bowl. Pour over almond, stir and serve.

Cauliflower Scramble

Serves: 4
Time: 15 minutes

Ingredients:

½ head cauliflower, cut into florets
2 garlic cloves, minced
1 red bell pepper, sliced
1 onion, chopped
4oz. whole mushrooms
1 tablespoon water
1 teaspoon turmeric
½ teaspoon black pepper, ground
Salt – to taste

Directions:

Cook the mushrooms, onion, and bell pepper in a skillet. Cook with 1 tablespoon water until veggies are tender. Add more water if needed to prevent sticking.

Add the cauliflower and cook until tender. Season to taste and add turmeric, garlic, and

black pepper. Cook for 5 minutes more, stirring
and serve after.

Apple Pecan Smoothie

Serves: 1
Time: 5 minutes

Ingredients:
1 cup almond milk
1 cup baby spinach
1 apple, sliced
½ avocado
2 plums
1 tablespoon pecans
1 teaspoon lemon zest

Directions:

Place pecans and milk in food processor. Pulse
until you have pecan milk.
Strain the milk and remove the pecans.

Pour milk back in the cleaned food processor
and add the rest of ingredients.
Pulse again until well combined.

Serve in a tall glass then sprinkle with some
pecans.

Breakfast Savory Cakes

Serves: 4
Time: 15 minutes

Ingredients:

1 cup whole wheat flour
½ cup corn meal
1 cup almond milk, unsweetened
1 green bell pepper, chopped
6oz. corn kernels, fresh
4 green onions, chopped
2 tablespoons avocado, mashed
½ teaspoon salt
¾ cup black beans, cooked

Directions:

Preheat oven to 200°F.

In a large bowl, combine whole-wheat flour,
corn meal, and salt. Make a well in the center
and pour in the almond milk. Stir until just
combined; stir in the corn kernels, black beans,
bell pepper, mashed avocado and green onions
until mixed well.

Heat a large non-stick skillet with 1 teaspoon
water; spoon ¼ cup of batter and place in the

skillet. Cook until underside is crisp, for 4 minutes. Flip the pancakes and cook for 4 minutes. Serve while still hot.

Quinoa Fruity Bowl

Serves: 2
Time: 15 minutes

Ingredients:

1 cup quinoa
½ cup soy milk
1 tablespoon flax seed meal
1 banana, sliced
2 tablespoons cranberries, dried
½ cup blueberries
¼ cup walnuts

Directions:

Place quinoa, banana, cranberries, blueberries, and flax meal in saucepot and cover with water; bring to simmer and remove from the heat. Cover and place aside until liquid is absorbed.

Transfer the quinoa in a bowl; pour the soy milk and serve.

Banana Pancakes

Serves: 5 pancakes
Time: 15 minutes

Ingredients:

1 cup whole wheat flour
1 teaspoon baking soda, aluminum-free
½ tablespoon chia seeds, ground
½ tablespoon water
1 cup soy milk
½ cup sparkling water
¾ cup blueberries, fresh
1 banana

Directions:

Combine the water and chia seeds in a bowl; place aside.

In a large bowl combine the wheat flour, baking soda and chia seeds mix.

Mash the banana in a separate bowl. Stir in the soy milk and sparkling water; mix until smooth. Fold the mixture into flour mixture then stir to combine.

Heat a non-stick skillet over medium-high heat; pour ¼ cup batter into skillet and flatten with back of the spoon. Sprinkle with blueberries and cook until bubbles appear. Flip and cook for 1-2 minutes. Repeat with remaining batter.

Serve the pancakes while still hot.

Blueberry Smoothie

Serves: 1
Time: 5 minutes

Ingredients:

½ cup blueberries
½ cup coconut milk
½ cup oats
1 tablespoon almond butter
½ cup water
½ teaspoon cinnamon

Directions:

Place the oats in a blender; pulse few times. Add the water and pulse again; allow to rest for 2 minutes.

Add remaining ingredients and pulse until smooth.

Potato Oven Pancakes

Yields: 20 mini pancakes
Time: 30 minutes

Ingredients:

2 russet potatoes, peeled, grated
½ cup whole-wheat flour
1 large zucchini, grated
½ onion, minced
1 teaspoon baking powder, aluminum free
2 teaspoons marjoram, dried
½ teaspoon black pepper

Directions:

Preheat oven to 425°F and line baking sheet with parchment paper.

Press the veggies, both potatoes and zucchinis to remove excess liquid. Place in a bowl and stir to combine.

In a separate bowl, combine the whole wheat flour with marjoram, baking soda and pepper.

Fold in the zucchini-potato mix and stir using wooden spoon.

Scoop ¼ cup of mixture and form into ball; flatten slightly with hands and place onto prepared baking sheet, leaving 1-inch space between. Bake the pancakes for 12 minutes, flip, and bake for 12 minutes more. Serve after with desired topping, like salsa.

100% Banana Muffins

Serves: 12 muffins
Time: 40 minutes

Ingredients:

4 bananas
1 teaspoon cinnamon
2 cups oats, ground into flour
½ cup water
2 tablespoons flax seeds, ground
½ tablespoon baking powder, aluminum-free
½ teaspoon baking soda, aluminum-free
½ tablespoon apple cider vinegar
½ cup applesauce, organic (just bake apples and mash)

Directions:

Preheat oven to 350F and line 12-hole muffin tin with paper cases.

Grind oats in food processor until you have a flour; add cinnamon, baking powder and soda. Pulse to combine.

Add remaining ingredients and pulse until combined; do not overmix. Spoon the batter into prepared muffin tin and bake in preheated oven for 20-22 minutes or until firm to touch. Place on wire rack to cool slightly before removing and serving.

Strawberry-Beet Smoothie

Serves: 1
Time: 5 minutes

Ingredients:

8oz. coconut water
¼ cup old-fashioned oats
10 strawberries
½ cup beets, chopped
¼ avocado, peeled, stoned

Directions:

Place the oats in blender and pulse until finely ground

Add coconut water and pulse for 10 seconds; allow to rest for 2 minutes.

Add remaining ingredients and pulse until blended and smooth.

Serve.

Veggie Breakfast Bowl

Serves: 4
Time: 20 minutes

Ingredients:

1 cup quinoa, cooked
1 onion, diced
1 cup baby spinach
1 tablespoon water
Salt and pepper, to taste
2 avocados, sliced
1 cup tomatoes, chopped

Directions:

Cook onions with 1 tablespoon water for 5 minutes over medium-high heat,

Add the tomatoes and cook for 5 minutes more over medium heat.

Toss in the spinach and season to taste. When the spinach is wilted, stir in the cooked quinoa and remove from the heat.

Divide the quinoa among four bowls and top with sliced avocado.

Banana Breakfast Cookies

Yields: 12 cookies
Time: 15 minutes

Ingredients:

2 ½ bananas, ripe
1 cup rolled oats
¼ cup walnuts, chopped
1 pinch cinnamon

Directions:

Preheat oven to 350°F and line baking sheet with parchment paper.

Mash bananas in a bowl; stir in the rolled oats, walnuts, and cinnamon.

Drop the mixture by spoonful onto baking sheet.

Bake the cookies for 15 minutes. Once baked place onto a wire rack and allow to cool.

Fig Smoothie

Serves: 1
Time: 5 minutes

Ingredients:

2 figs, fresh, timed, quartered
6 strawberries. Fresh
½ banana, sliced
1 cup almond milk
1 teaspoon cinnamon
1 tablespoon chia seeds
Directions:

Combine all the ingredients in a blender.

Process until smooth.

Serve immediately.

Baked Fruity Oatmeal

Serves: 4
Time: 50 minutes

Ingredients:

1 cup rolled oats
1 tablespoon chopped pecans
2 tablespoons chopped dried apricots

1 cup almond milk, unsweetened
2 tablespoons chopped dried plums
¼ cup + 1 tablespoon baked purred apple or unsweetened apple sauce
½ teaspoon ground cinnamon

Directions:

Preheat oven to 350°F and prepare 6x6-inch baking pan.

Place all listed ingredients by order in a bowl.

Stir well to combine and transfer into prepared pan.

Bake the prepared mixture for 40 minutes or until slightly brown on top.

Set on wire rack to cool before slicing and serving.

Lunch Recipes

Potato Soup

Serves: 4
Time: 35 minutes

Ingredients:

3 cups water
½ teaspoon ground sea salt
4 cups potatoes, peeled and cubed
½ cup almond milk
2 garlic cloves, minced
1 teaspoon dried parsley
1 cup carrots, chopped
1 cup celery, chopped
Small pinch black pepper
½ teaspoon thyme
½ small onion, chopped

Directions:

Add celery, carrots, and onion in a saucepan with 2 tablespoons water; cook until tender.

Add garlic and cook for 1 minute further.

Pour in the remaining water and add potatoes, spices, and herbs.

Reduce heat to medium-low, stir and simmer for 30 minutes or until potatoes are tender.

Remove from the heat and transfer half of the potatoes into food processor.

Pulse until smooth and place in the soup.

Stir in almond milk and set back over heat until heated through.

Serve while still hot.

Oven Baked Mexican Bean Burgers

Serves: 4
Time: 20 minutes

Ingredients:

¼ cup whole wheat flour
8 oz. kidney beans, drained and mashed
2 tablespoons almond flour
1 small carrot, grated
Salt and pepper
½ cup finely chopped onion
2 teaspoons chili powder

Directions:

Place all ingredients in a bowl, except flour.

Stir well and gradually add flour. Stir again until flour is well incorporated.

Preheat oven to 450∘F and line baking sheet with parchment paper.

For patties from prepared mixture and arrange onto baking sheet.

Bake for 10-12 minutes or until firm and nicely brown.

Serve with salad or salsa while still hot.

Portabella "Steaks" And Veggies

Serves: 4
Time: 20 minutes

Ingredients:

4 portabella mushrooms
1 cup sliced bell pepper
1 cup carrot, cut into sticks
4 garlic cloves, thinly sliced
½ teaspoon crushed red pepper
½ teaspoon salt
1 cup broccoli florets
½ cup finely chopped onions

1 teaspoon ginger

Directions:

Place the mushrooms in a bowl and pour over some water; sprinkle with ginger and place aside for 15 minutes.

Heat 1 tablespoon water in a sauce pot over medium heat and add the onion.
Cook onions until soft then add prepared veggies.

Cook, covered for 8-10 minutes or until veggies are tender.

Heat separate skillet over medium-high heat and when hot add portabella mushrooms.

Cook until portabella are cooked, 3 minutes per side.

Serve while still hot with vegetables on top.

White Bean-Quinoa Lunch Salad

Serves: 4
Time: 15 minutes

Ingredients:

2 cups cooked quinoa

2 cups cooked white beans
1 scallion, chopped
2 tablespoons chopped fresh parsley
1 red bell pepper, diced
Salt and pepper – to taste
3 tablespoons lemon juice
1 tablespoon avocado, mashed
1 tablespoon water
1 teaspoon marjoram, dried

Directions:

In a large mixing bowl, combine quinoa, white beans, bell pepper, scallions, and season with salt and pepper.

Combine avocado, lemon juice, marjoram and water in a bowl; season and drizzle over prepared salad.

Serve immediately.

String Beans With Sesame

Serves: 2
Time: 15 minutes

Ingredients:

2 cups string beans, cut into 2-inch pieces
2 garlic cloves, minced

1 tablespoon water
Salt and pepper
1 tablespoon sesame seeds
2 dried chili peppers, sliced

Directions:

Blanche string beans in large pot of salted water for 3 minutes over medium-high heat.

Drain and set on kitchen towel to dry.

Heat 1 tablespoon water add garlic, sesame and chili pepper. Cook for 30 seconds.

Add cooked beans and stir until well coated.

Transfer to a plate and serve.

Veggie Slow Cooker Goulas

Serves: 8
Time: 6 hours

Ingredients:

4 tomatoes, cut into wedges
3 garlic cloves, chopped
1 jalapeno pepper, diced
½ bunch parsley, chopped
1 tablespoon smoked paprika

2 onions, sliced into half moons

2 bay leaves

1 lb. green beans, trimmed and chopped into ½-inch pieces

1 cup corn

4 cups water

4 tablespoons vinegar

2 green bell peppers, chopped

2 red bell peppers, chopped

Salt and pepper – to taste

Directions:

Place spices, water, veggies, and vinegar in a slow cooker.

Cover and cook on low for 6 hours.

Serve while still hot

Squash And Coconut Slow-Cooker Curry

Serves: 4
Time: 6 hours

Ingredients:

½ cup onion, diced

1 garlic clove, minced

1 tomato, diced

1 ½ cup water

7 oz. coconut milk

¾ cup peas

1 ½ tablespoons mild curry

¾ cup black soy beans, soaked in water for 24 hours

1 ¼ cups butternut squash, peeled and cubed into 1-inch cubes

½ cup chopped kale

½ teaspoon salt

1 tablespoon chopped cilantro

Directions:

Add all ingredients in slow cooker, except kale and peas.

Stir well, cover, and cook on high for 6 hours.

Around 30 minutes before serving add in the fresh peas and kale.

Give it a stir and continue cooking for those 30 minutes.

Serve while still hot with some brown rice garnished with cilantro.

Yellow Split Pea Stew

Serves: 4
Time: 50 minutes

Ingredients:

2 cups water + 1 ½ tablespoons, divided
¾ cup split yellow peas
1 large garlic clove, minced
½-inch ginger, grated
¾ teaspoon salt
¼ teaspoon turmeric
½ small onion, chopped

Directions:

Place 2 cups water and peas in a medium sized saucepan.

Heat over high heat and bring to boil.

Reduce heat to medium and cook split peas until tender, for 30 minutes.

Meanwhile heat remaining water in skillet. Add onions and cook for 5 minutes or until tender. Add garlic, turmeric and ginger; cook for 2 minutes or until fragrant.

Add mixture to the cooked peas and stir well. Season additionally with salt and pepper.

Oven Baked Cauliflower Steaks

Serves: 4
Time: 45 minutes

Ingredients:

1 head cauliflower, cut into steaks
2 tablespoons applesauce, unsweetened
Salt and pepper
1 teaspoon fennel seeds

Directions:

Preheat oven to 420F and line baking tray with parchment paper.

Place cauliflower steaks on baking sheet and brush with applesauce. Season with salt and pepper and sprinkle with fennel seeds.

Bake for 35-40 minutes or until cabbage is tender and edges are golden.

Serve when cooled slightly.

Green Beans And Pine Nuts

Serves: 4
Time: 15 minutes

Ingredients:

1 lb. green beans, cut into ½.inch pieces
¼ cup pine nuts
1 tablespoon lime juice
Salt and pepper, to taste

Directions:

Cook beans in large pot of salted water for 5 minutes and drain well.

Meanwhile heat a non-stick skillet and add the pine nuts; toast dry for few minutes or until fragrant.

Stir the beans with pine nuts and transfer to a bowl.

Drizzle with lemon juice and season to taste.

Toss to combine and serve.

Rice and Bean Casserole

Serves: 4
Time: 70 minutes

Ingredients:

2 cups brown rice, uncooked

15 oz. can of red kidney beans, drained and rinsed

15 oz. can of black beans, drained and rinsed

15 oz. can of garbanzo beans, drained and rinsed

4 oz. can of mild chilies, drained

1 cup onion, chopped

14 oz. tomatoes, pureed

10 oz. green peas

1 cup corn

3 – 3 ½ cups water

Directions:

Preheat oven to 350°F.

Heat 1 tablespoon water in cooking pot or Dutch oven over medium-high heat and add onion. Cook for 5 minutes or until tender.

Add rice and stir while cooking until slightly opaque.

Add tomatoes, beans, chilies, and water. Bring mixture to boil over high heat.

Cover tightly and place in the oven. Cook for 60 minutes or until liquid is absorbed and rice tender.

Add peas and corn and season according to your desire. Place back in the oven to reheat.

Serve while still hot.

Roasted Lunch Bowl

Serves: 4
Time: 45 minutes

Ingredients:

1 head broccoli, cut into florets
1 head cauliflower, cut into florets
10oz. cannellini beans, cooked
1 handful radishes, halved
¼ cup tahini
2 tablespoons water
Juice of 1 lemon
2 garlic cloves, minced
1 cup quinoa, cooked
Salt and pepper, to taste

Directions:

Prepare the dressing; in a food processor combine the lemon juice, garlic, tahini, water, and beans. Season to taste and process until smooth. Place aside.
Preheat oven to 400F. In a large bowl, combine the broccoli, cauliflower, and radishes. Season with salt and pepper and sprinkle with water.

Toss to coat and spread over baking sheet.
Roast for 30-40 minutes, stirring once.
Serve roasted veggies over cooked quinoa and
pour over prepared dressing. Serve after.

Falafel Wrap

Serves: 4
Time: 30 minutes

Ingredients:

1lb. chickpeas, cooked
1 tablespoon tahini
1 garlic clove, minced
1 teaspoon smoked paprika
1 teaspoon coriander, ground
2 tablespoons whole-wheat flour
1 onion, minced
2 tablespoons parsley, freshly chopped
1 tablespoon water
4 whole-wheat wraps
Salt and pepper, to taste

Directions:

Mash cooked chickpeas in a bowl. Place aside.

Cook onion and garlic with water in skillet over
medium-high heat.

Add paprika, coriander and cook for 30 seconds more. Remove from the heat.

Transfer onion mixture in a bowl with chickpeas. Add the parsley, flour, tahini, and season to taste. Mix until combined and form balls from the prepared mixture.

Arrange falafel balls onto a baking sheet, brush with water and bake for 15 minutes at 375°F.

Once browned remove from the heat place on top of whole-wheat tortilla wraps. You can add some fresh salad before wrapping and serving.

Bean And Vegetable Chili

Serves: 6
Time: 25 minutes

Ingredients:

1 onion, chopped
14oz. tomatoes, pureed
3 cups pinto beans, cooked
2 teaspoons chili powder
1 teaspoon cumin
1 ½ cups corn kernels, fresh
1 green bell pepper, sliced
1 ½ cups zucchini, diced
¼ teaspoon salt

2 garlic cloves, minced

Directions:

In a cooking pan, cook the onion, garlic and bell pepper with 1 tablespoon water, over medium heat until tender.

Add the beans, puree tomatoes, and seasonings. Bring to boil and reduce heat; simmer for 10 minutes. Stir in the corn and zucchinis and continue cooking for 7-8 minutes or until zucchinis are tender.

Serve while still hot.

Quinoa Stuffed Tomatoes

Serves: 4
Time: 40 minutes

Ingredients:

4 large tomatoes
1 cup corn kernels
2 garlic cloves, minced
½ onion, diced
2 cups black beans, cooked
2 cups quinoa, cooked
½ yellow bell pepper, chopped
Salt and pepper, to taste

½ tablespoon basil, fresh, chopped

Directions:

Preheat oven to 350∘F.

Cut the tops of tomatoes and scoop out the flesh.

Place the onion and bell pepper in a cooking pan; cook over medium heat with 1-2 tablespoons of water until veggies are tender.

Add garlic and cook for 2 minutes more. Add the cooked beans, quinoa, and corn. Season with salt and pepper and cook for 5 minutes. Stuff the prepared tomatoes with prepared mixture. Transfer the tomatoes onto baking dish and bake for 30 minutes, covered with aluminum foil. Remove and serve while still hot.

Bean Bites

Serves: 4
Time: 25 minutes

Ingredients:

15oz. kidney beans, cooked
1 garlic clove, minced
½ onion, minced

½ tablespoon basil, fresh chopped

1 teaspoon thyme, dried

1 teaspoon oregano, dried

1 tablespoon chili powder

6 tablespoons oats, soaked in water for 3 hours drained

1 cup broccoli florets, chopped

Directions:

Preheat oven to 350°F and line 8-hole muffin with paper cases.

Mash beans in a bowl with fork or potato masher.

Add in remaining ingredients and stir to combine.

Spoon the mixture into paper cases and bake for 20 minutes.

Place on a wire rack to cool for 5 minutes before removing from the tin and serving.

Broccoli Soup

Serves: 6
Time: 30 minutes

Ingredients:

1 ½ lb. Yukon gold potatoes, peeled, cut into
chunks
2 garlic cloves, minced
1 onion, chopped
1 ½ lb. broccoli, coarsely chopped
3 leaves Swiss chard, trimmed and coarsely
chopped
Salt and pepper, to taste
1 sprig thyme, fresh
6 cups water

Directions:

Cook the onion with 1 tablespoon water in
saucepan over medium-high heat until tender.

Add the garlic and cook for 1 minute. Add the
potatoes, thyme, water, and season to taste.

Bring to boil and reduce the heat then add the
broccoli. Cook, covered for 10-12 minutes or
until potatoes are tender.

Stir in the Swiss chard and cook for 5 minutes. Remove from the heat and let it stand for 5 minutes. Puree the soup using immersion blender and adjust the seasoning.

Vegetable Stew

Serves: 6
Time: 50 minutes

Ingredients:

1lb. butternut squash
2 teaspoons cumin, ground
1 tablespoon sweet paprika
8 cups water
1 turnip, peeled and cut into ½-inch pieces
15oz. tomatoes, pureed
2 tablespoons mint, chopped
½ cup cilantro, fresh, chopped
2 celery stalks, chopped
1 onion, peeled, chopped
2 carrots, peeled, chopped
2 cups chickpeas, cooked
2 cloves garlic, minced
Salt and pepper, to taste

Directions:

Cook the onion, carrots, and celery in saucepan with 1-2 tablespoons water until tender, over medium-high heat.

Add the garlic, cumin, paprika and cook for 3 minutes. Add the water, squash, chickpeas, turnip, potato, and tomatoes. Bring to boil over high heat.

Reduce heat to low and simmer for 25 minutes; stir in the herbs and cook for 10 minutes. Serve while still hot.

Quinoa Curry Bowl

Serves: 4
Time: 15 minutes

Ingredients:

¾ cup quinoa
1 ½ teaspoons curry powder
1 tablespoon ginger, minced
2 tablespoons tahini
8oz. green snap beans
4oz. broccoli florets
4oz. cauliflower florets
4 garlic cloves, minced
1 ½ cups water
Salt and pepper, to taste

Directions:

In a saucepan combine the water, quinoa and ½ curry powder. Bring to boil and reduce heat; simmer for 15 minutes, covered.

Meanwhile, cook the green beans, broccoli, and cauliflower in a skillet. Cook with 2-3 tablespoons of water or until tender. You can also steam the veggies.

Once the veggies are cooked stir in the remaining powder, garlic, and ginger. Season to taste and cook for 2 minutes.

Remove from the heat and stir in the tahini. Add water if needed to thin.

Flake the quinoa with fork and combine with veggies. Toss to combine and serve. Adjust the seasoning before serving.

Rainbow Burgers

Serves: 8 burgers
Time: 40 minutes

Ingredients:

15oz. kidney beans, cooked
½ cup parley flour
2 cups brown rice, cooked

½ cup cornmeal

2 garlic cloves, minced

1 cup onion, minced

1 cup tomato, diced

1 cup broccoli florets

½ cup corn kernels

Salt and pepper, to taste

2 teaspoons thyme, dried

1 teaspoon cumin, ground

Directions:

Preheat oven to 350°F and line 2 baking sheets with parchment paper.

In a large bowl, combine the rice, beans, cornmeal, barley flour, onion, garlic, thyme, and cumin. Stir and squish all with clean hands.

Add the tomato, corn, and broccoli. Season to taste and squish again.

Scoop 1 cup of the mixture and form a ball from the mixture. Place onto baking sheet and flatten to ½ inch thick.

Bake burgers for 20 minutes in preheated oven; remove, flip and cook for 20 minutes more.

Serve with fresh salad and whole-wheat bun.

Veggie Based Loaf

Serves: 4
Time: 60 minutes

Ingredients:

15oz. black beans, cooked
1 carrot, peeled, shredded
1 cup brown mushrooms, chopped
1 cup quinoa, cooked
3 tablespoons whole-wheat flour
5 tablespoons tomato, pureed
2 teaspoons basil, dried
2 teaspoons oregano, dried
2 teaspoons marjoram, dried
2 celery stalks, shredded
1 onion, chopped finely
Salt and pepper, to taste

Directions:

Preheat oven to 350°F and prepare 8-inch non-stick loaf pan.

Mash beans in a bowl using potato masher and add remaining ingredients, reserving 1 tablespoon pureed tomato. Season to taste.

Mix well and transfer into loaf pan. Brush with reserved tomato puree.

Bake for 50-55 minutes until firm and brown outside.

Allow to cool for 20 minutes before removing from the pan and serving.

Dinner Recipes

Mediterranean Couscous

Serves: 4
Time: 20 minutes

Ingredients:

1 cup vegetable stock, homemade
¾ cup whole-wheat couscous, uncooked
1 small cucumber, unpeeled but properly washed, diced
1/8 teaspoon salt
3 medium tomatoes, diced and seeded
2 tablespoons water
2 tablespoons tahini
2 tablespoons lemon juice
4 medium green onions, chopped
1 tablespoon chopped cilantro

Directions:

In a 2-quart sauce pan heat stock over high heat and bring to boil.

Stir in couscous and remove from the heat. Let it stand for 5 minutes.

In a large bowl, combine cucumber, tomatoes, onions and cilantro then add couscous.

In small bowl whisk tahini, water, lemon juice and salt. Pour over prepared couscous and veggies. Toss to combine and serve.

Sweet Potato Burgers

Serves: 4
Time: 30 minutes

Ingredients:

1 ½ cups sweet potatoes, cooked with skin
¼ cup fresh corn
8 oz. black beans, cooked
¼ teaspoon chili powder
½ teaspoon cumin
¼ cup chopped onion
3 tablespoons rolled oats
1 tablespoon sunflower seeds
¼ teaspoon salt
1 garlic clove, minced
¼ cup cooked quinoa
½ teaspoon dried basil

Directions:

Preheat oven to 350∘F and line baking sheet with parchment paper.

Mash half of the beans, but leave some chunks.

Add in the rest of beans and stir to combine.

In a large bowl, gently mash the sweet potatoes; stir in spices and dried basil.

Add oats, corn, black beans, quinoa, sunflower seeds, garlic, and onion and stir well to combine.

Form balls from the mixture and flatten to ½-inch thick patties.

Arrange patties onto prepared baking sheet and bake in preheated oven for 15 minutes per side.

Remove and serve with some fresh buns and fresh sliced avocado or peppers.

Red Lentil Curry

Serves: 4
Time: 30 minutes

Ingredients:

1 cup red lentils
½ teaspoon chili powder
½ teaspoon ground cumin
½ teaspoon salt
½ teaspoon minced garlic
½ tablespoon curry powder

½ teaspoon ground turmeric
½ cup onion, chopped
½ tablespoon water
1 tablespoon curry paste
½ teaspoon minced ginger
7 oz. tomatoes, pureed in blender

Directions:

Wash lentils under cold water and place in a pot. Add enough water around 2 cups and heat over medium-high heat.

Cover and bring lentils to simmer. Reduce heat to medium and simmer until tender. Add more water if necessary.

Meanwhile in a large skillet heat ½ tablespoon water. Add onions and cook over medium-low heat for 10 minutes or until caramelized.

Combine curry paste, curry powder, and remaining spices in mixing bowl.

When the onions are cooked, add the curry mixture to the onions and cook over high heat, stirring constantly for 1-2 minutes.

Stir in the tomato puree and reduce heat. Simmer until lentils are ready.

Drain the lentils briefly and mix the curry base in.

Serve while still hot garnished with fresh chopped cilantro.

"Meatballs" Without Meat

Serves: 4
Time: 60 minutes

Ingredients:

¼ cup dried lentils
¾ cup water
¼ teaspoon salt
¼ teaspoon garlic
1 tablespoon flax seeds meal
1 tablespoon chopped walnuts
5 oz. frozen chopped spinach, thawed and pat dry
¼ cup brown rice flour
½ teaspoon dried basil
1 small garlic clove, minced
½ cup sliced mushrooms

Directions:

Place lentils and water in medium sized sauce pan and bring to boil over high heat.

Reduce heat to medium-low and add garlic and half of the onion.

Cover and simmer for 40-45 minutes.

Preheat oven to 350°F and brush baking tray with some olive oil.

Cook spinach, mushrooms, and remaining onion in skillet with 1-2 tablespoons water.

Cook for 5 minutes stirring frequently.

When lentils are done, drain and add to the spinach mixture. Add rice flour, walnuts, basil, and spices.

Stir well and transfer to food processor. Blend for 10 seconds or until almost smooth.

Form "meatballs" from the mixture and arrange onto prepared tray.

Bake for 25-30 minutes. Set on wire rack to cool slightly before serving. Serve with fresh homemade tomato sauce.

Spring Quinoa

Serves: 4
Time: 35 minutes

Ingredients:

1/3 cup quinoa
¾ cup water
Small pinch salt
1/3 cup chopped asparagus
1/3 cup chopped red bell peppers
1 ½ tablespoons pine nuts
1 small red onion, diced
1/3 cup chopped tomatoes, seeded
1 tablespoon chopped fresh parsley
1 garlic clove, minced
½ teaspoon dried oregano

Directions:

Rinse quinoa and place in a sauce pan.

Add water and bring to boil over high heat.

Reduce heat to low and simmer for 20 minutes or until nearly all liquid is absorbed.

Cook onions with 1 tablespoon water in skillet over medium-high heat until tender. Add garlic and cook further for 1 minute or until fragrant.

Add remaining veggies, additional water and cook over low heat for 7 minutes.

Add cooked quinoa to the skillet and stir in parsley, pine nuts, and oregano.

Stir well and serve while still hot.

Lettuce Wraps

Serves: 4
Time: 10 minutes

Ingredients:

1 cup hummus
½ cup sliced cucumber
8 romaine lettuce leaves
½ cup zucchini, chopped
½ cup shredded carrots
1 small bell pepper, sliced into thin stripes
Squeeze of fresh lemon juice.

Directions:

Spread 2 tablespoon of hummus over lettuce leaves and sprinkle with few drops of lemon juice.

Top with carrots, cucumbers, zucchinis, and pepper.

Roll up like tortilla and serve.

Veggie Pizza

Serves: 4
Time: 40 minutes

Ingredients:

1 cup warm water
2 ½ cups whole wheat flour
1 teaspoon salt
2 tablespoons flaxseed meal
1 cup tomatoes, pureed
1 onion, sliced into thin rounds
1 cup sliced mushrooms
1 green bell pepper, sliced
½ cup raw macadamia nuts

Directions:

Preheat oven to 450°F.

Mix flour, salt, flaxseeds and water in food processor. Pulse until dough forms.

Turn dough onto floured surface and knead several times with hands.

Roll the dough with floured rolling pin to 12-inch circle and place onto pizza stone or onto baking sheet sprinkled with some whole-wheat flour.

Bake for 10 minutes and remove from the oven; set on wire rack.

Spread tomato sauce on top of baked crust and top with mushrooms, onion, and bell pepper.

Bake for 20 minutes and remove from oven.

Meanwhile process macadamia nuts in food processor and sprinkle on top of prepared pizza.

Slice and serve.

Rice and Tahini Cakes

Serves: 4
Time: 25 minutes

Ingredients:

1 tablespoon tahini
1 ½ cups cooked brown rice
2 tablespoons chopped spring onions
2 tablespoons ground old fashioned oats
1 teaspoon dried parsley

Directions:

Combine all ingredients in a bowl. Stir well.

Heat olive oil in large skillet over medium-high heat.

Form cakes from the prepared mixture, around 1/3 cup.

Preheat oven to 350°F and line baking sheet with parchment paper. Arrange cakes onto baking sheet and bake for 15-20 minutes or until browned. Serve while still hot with fresh salad.

Cauliflower Rice With Zucchinis

Serves: 2
Time: 15 minutes

Ingredients:

2 cups cauliflower "rice" (simply process cauliflower to get 2 cups), steamed
1 medium zucchini, cut into ½-inch cubes
½ teaspoon chili powder
¼ teaspoon ground cumin
Salt and pepper
½ tablespoon lemon juice
2 tablespoons chopped mint
1 small onion, chopped
2 garlic cloves, minced
1 tablespoon water

Directions:

Heat a large non-stick skillet over medium heat. Cook onion with water until tender, for 5 minutes.

Add garlic and cook for 30 seconds.

Add zucchinis; cook for 5 minutes, or until just tender.

Reduce heat to low and stir in the spices; season with salt and pepper, to taste.

Add steamed cauliflower "rice" and toss to combine well.

Set aside for 5 minutes before serving.

Soy Beans Salad With Asparagus And Dill

Serves: 2
Time: 10 minutes

Ingredients:

½ cup can black soy beans, rinsed, drained
1 garlic clove, minced
¼ cup diced tomatoes
½ cup diced asparagus
2 tablespoons lemon juice

1 tablespoon fresh dill, chopped
1 tablespoon water
2 tablespoons pureed avocado
Freshly ground salt

Directions:

Place asparagus in a large pot and cover with water. Simmer for 2 minutes or until crisp-tender. Drain and place in a large bowl.

Add soy beans, tomato, and dill. Combine water, avocado puree, and lemon juice in another bowl; drizzle over salad.

Season with salt and toss to combine. Serve in a small bowls

Soy Bean And Spinach Slow-Cooker Enchiladas

Serves: 8
Time: 3 hours

Ingredients:

10 oz. chopped spinach
15 oz. soybeans, cooked rinsed and drained (or black beans)
½ teaspoon ground cumin
6 cups chopped lettuce

½ cup grape tomatoes, halved
½ cucumber, halved and sliced
3 tablespoons lime juice, fresh
3 cups salsa
8 whole-wheat tortillas, homemade
½ cup cashew halves - -processed in a blender
for 15 seconds

Directions:

In a medium bowl, mash half of the soybeans.
Add cumin, spinach, ¼ cup processed cashews,
remaining soybeans, salt, and pepper; stir to
combine.

Spread 1 cup salsa in the bottom of 4 quart
slow cooker.

Divide bean mixture evenly between whole-
wheat tortillas and place them seam side down
on top of salsa and pour over remaining salsa
and cashews.

Cover and cook on low for 3 hours.

Combine lettuce, lime juice, salt and pepper in
a bowl; toss to combine.

Serve with prepared enchiladas.

Braised Cabbage with Raisins

Serves: 4
Time: 30 minutes

Ingredients:

1 cabbage, red, medium size, sliced thinly
2 shallots, thinly sliced
1 ½ teaspoons salt
2 tablespoons lemon juice
1/3 cup raisins
Salt and pepper
2 teaspoons cider vinegar
1 tablespoon water

Directions:

Heat water in non-stick pan and when hot and cabbage and shallots.

Cook, stirring occasionally for 15 minutes.

Stir in remaining ingredients, except raisins and season with salt and pepper.

Cook further for 12 minutes and stir in raisins.

Serve while still hot.

Spicy Tomato and Basil Soup

Serves: 4
Time: 45 minutes

Ingredients:

1 ½ tablespoons water
1 cup onion, chopped
28 oz. fresh tomatoes, chopped
2-3 cups water
1 garlic clove, crushed
1 teaspoon cayenne pepper
½ teaspoon chili flakes
5 basil leaves, chopped
1 cup carrots, grated
¾ cup fresh orange juice
½ cup mushrooms, pureed

Directions:

Heat 1 tablespoon water in a medium-sized pot over medium-high heat. Add onions, grated carrots, and garlic. Cook for 10-12 minutes stirring occasionally.

Add the tomatoes, orange juice, and water. Bring to boil and reduce heat to medium. Add chopped basil and spices.

Let it simmer for 25-30 minutes or until tomatoes are nicely tender.

Remove the soup from the heat and using hand blender or food processor puree the tomatoes.

Stir in pureed mushrooms and simmer for 5 more minutes.

Serve while still hot and garnish with fresh basil.

Curry Zucchini Soup

Serves: 6
Time: 30 minutes

Ingredients:

6 cups diced zucchinis
1 tablespoon water
2 garlic cloves, minced
1 cup yellow onion, chopped
2 teaspoons mild curry
6 cups vegetable stock, homemade
¼ cup basmati rice
Salt and pepper
¼ teaspoon cayenne pepper
2 tablespoons fresh lime juice
To garnish:
2 tablespoons fresh chopped chives

Directions:

Heat 1 tablespoons water in medium-sized pot and add chopped onion.

Cook for 5 minutes or until tender, stirring occasionally.

Add zucchinis, garlic and season with salt and pepper; stir well and cook for 1 minute or until garlic is very fragrant.

Add the curry powder, cayenne pepper, vegetable stock and stir well.

Bring to boil over high heat and reduce heat then cover and simmer for 30 minutes.

Set aside to cool slightly and using immersion blender puree the soup in batches.

Return to the pot and heat through; add lime juice and serve while still hot, with chives on top.

Conclusion

I hope you found this book helpful and that you will improve your eating habits, because feeding our body with the right foods is the best way to stay fit and healthy.